Useful Diagnos

Anass M. Abbas Omer

Useful Diagnostic Techniques in Oral Cytopathology

Patients Care and Promising Career in Laboratory
Medicine and Medical Technology with Young
Medical Scientists

LAP LAMBERT Academic Publishing

Imprint
Any brand names and product names mentioned in this book are subject to
trademark, brand or patent protection and are trademarks or registered
trademarks of their respective holders. The use of brand names, product
names, common names, trade names, product descriptions etc. even without
a particular marking in this work is in no way to be construed to mean that
such names may be regarded as unrestricted in respect of trademark and
brand protection legislation and could thus be used by anyone.

Cover image: www.ingimage.com

Publisher:
LAP LAMBERT Academic Publishing
is a trademark of
International Book Market Service Ltd., member of OmniScriptum Publishing
Group
17 Meldrum Street, Beau Bassin 71504, Mauritius

Printed at: see last page
ISBN: 978-613-9-45660-4

Useful Diagnostic Cytological Techniques in Oral Cytopathology; Applied in the Assessment of Cellular Proliferative Activity in Oral Epithelium among Toombak Users

Submitted by:

Dr.Anass M. Abbas, MIBMS (UK), Ph.D.

-Ass.Professor of Laboratory Medicine (Histopathology-Cytopathology)
-Consultant Laboratory Medicine
-Research Associate in Cancer Pathology& Oncology
Department of Clinical Laboratory Sciences, CAMS, Jouf University, KSA
Medical Laboratory program, Alyarmouk Medical College, Sudan

DEDICATION

I dedicate this work to my father who encourages me to the road of success and happiness.

To my kind and lovely mother who taught me the meaning of life. To my Dear wife (Dr. Manar) who supported me brothers, sister, relatives and friends

ACKNOWLEDGEMENT

- My special thanks and appreciation to all of those who have helped me through their assistance and guidance in performing this work.

- I am indebted to my Dear teacher Prof.Hussain Gad Elkarim Ahmed for his sincere help and guidance.

- Also I would to thank the staff in the department of Histopathology and Cytology faculty of Medical Laboratory Sciences Alneelain University, Sudan. All thanks to our colleagues at the faculty of medical laboratory sciences Sudan University of science and technology. Special thanks to the department Clinical Laboratory Sciences, College of Appleid Medical Sciences, Jouf University, KSA.

Abstract

This is a retrospective case control cohort study aimed to compare the cytological Methods; papanicolaou stain, mean AgNOR counts, micronuclei frequency and 1% crystal violet stain which are Used in the Assessment of Cellular Proliferative Activity in the buccal mucosa of Toombak users and non-tobacco users. The smears were obtained from 210 participants of which two hundred apparently healthy individuals; one hundred were Toombak users (cases) the remaining hundred were non-tobacco users (controls) and ten patients with Oral Squamous Cell Carcinoma (OSCC), as an internal control, their ages ranging from 16 to 94 years with a mean age 33 years old. The mean age for the cases was (34 years); hence, the mean age for the controls was (32 years).

Cytological atypia was identified among four (4%) Toombak users and not found in control group, of the four cases with cytological atypia, only one case was identified with moderate degree of cytological atypia and the remaining three were categorized as having mild degree of cytological atypia (p< 0.04). Toombak dipping is a major factor for occurrence of the keratinization in the oral mucosa (P < 0.0001). In regard to the infections and inflammatory conditions, cases were more susceptible than control groups, erosions and exposure of oral mucosa to Toombak irritation are the major causative factors.

The mean AgNOR counts in the cases (2.423) was Statistically higher than control groups (1.303) (P < 0.0001). In regard to the mean of the micronuclei frequency per

4

1000 buccal cells, the micronuclei frequencies was higher in the cases group (1.026) than control group (0.356) (P < 0.0001). The mean of the AgNOR counts and micronuclei frequency was statistically increased with the prolonged and frequent use of Toombak (P < 0.001). However, there was increasing in the mean AgNOR counts in those snuffing large amount of Toombak per dip (relatively statistically significant; p<0.062).

The keratinization presence was associated with the increasing of the mean in the AgNOR counts and micronuclei frequency (p<0.0001). In regard to the presence of inflammation the AgNOR counts was statistically associated with the inflammation (p<0.006), hence, no evidence of relationship between inflammation presence and micronuclei frequency and the cytological atypia with inflammation presence. Increasing of the age in the study population was statistically associated with increasing of the proliferative markers (the mean AgNOR count and micronuclei frequency) and keratinization presence (p<0.001). Neither cases groups nor control groups were found with mitotic figures in 1% crystal violet stain method. This findings support that Toombak dipping is a high risk factor to increase the cellular proliferation in the oral mucosa and the cellular proliferative cytological methods are used as screening methods for Toombak users.

CHAPTER ONE

Introduction

No communicable diseases (NCDs) are the leading for the majority of global deaths, and worldwide cancer is expected to rank as the leading cause of death and the single most important barrier to increasing life expectancy in every country of the world. Globally the new cases and deaths from oral cancer is 92,887 (0.5) of the total cancer cases (Freddie, et al. 2018).All parts of the oral cavity are susceptible to cancer from tobacco smoking or chewing(snuffing), including the lip, tongue, palate, gum, and cheek. There exists today a need to identify biomarkers of oral cancer and their association with tobacco products. When compared with other body sites, the mouth offers a unique opportunity for defining biomarkers because the mouth permits noninvasive and repetitive examinations. Thirty percent to 80% of the malignancies of the oral cavity arise from premalignant lesions, such as leukoplakia, erythroplakia, and oral sub mucous fibrosis (Parkin, et al. 2002).

The most common type of cancer detection is a visual inspection of the mouth. But This, however has limitation. The cytological study of the cells in oral cavity is simple, rapid and non-invasive. So it's suitable for routine application in population screening programs, for early analysis of suspect lesions, and for pre-and post-treatment monitoring of confirmed malignant lesions (Taybos, 2003). Buccal cells are shed spontaneously (e.g., exfoliative cells) and daily from healthy buccal mucosa. In this respect, buccal cells are similar to cells shed in the vagina and harvested by scraping (i.e., Papanicolaou smear). The exfoliative buccal cells are end-stage cells of

6

differentiation and seldom display mitotic figures. Buccal cells can be collected from different sites of the mouth. These include the cheek, tongue, including the dorsal, lateral, and ventral surfaces, soft palate, hard palate, and oral pharynx—all of which are sites of oral cancer (Silverman, 2003). Diverse methods have been used successfully for harvesting buccal cells. These include scraping with a wood spatula, wood tongue depressor, cotton swab, short-bristle cytobrush, and toothbrush. Buccal cells assay used most frequently for tobacco-associated buccal cell changes that include micronuclei assay, changes in cell morphology and cellular proliferative activity. Clinical studies have correlated buccal cell changes with malignant tumors, and some oral oncologists have reported that the buccal cell changes are practical biomarkers. Summarily, the literature has established that buccal cells are useful not only for characterizing the molecular mechanisms underlying tobacco-associated oral cancers but also as exfoliative cells that express diverse changes that offer promise as candidate biomarkers for the early detection of oral cancer. It is envisioned, therefore, that cells of the mouth (buccal cells) will show progressive tobacco-induced changes, and that these alterations will precede and predict subsequent incipient (i.e., earlier than visible pathology) diseases of the lung (Shulman, et al. 2004).

The use of Toombak has been stated to play a major role in the etiology of oral cancer in the Sudan and is suspected to be associated with neoplasm of salivary glands. Toombak dippers develop a clinically and histologically characteristic lesion at the site of dipping. The risk for cancer of the oral cavity among Toombak users was high (RR 7.3-73.0-fold). The use of Toombak plays a significant role in etiology of oral squamous cell carcinomas (OSCCs), with the tobacco specific nitrosamines present in Toombak possibly acting as principal carcinogens (Ahmed and Mahgoob, 2007).

The Buccal Micronucleus assay is a minimally invasive method for studying DNA damage, chromosomal instability, cell death and the regenerative potential of human buccal mucosal tissue. This method is increasingly used in molecular epidemiological studies for investigating the impact of nutrition, lifestyle factors, genotoxin exposure and genotype on DNA damage, chromosome malsegregation and cell death. The biomarkers measured in this assay have been associated with increased risk of accelerated ageing, cancer and neurodegenerative diseases (Thomas, et al. 2007).

argyrophilic nucleolar organizer region (AgNOR) is silver staining procedure to observe the nucleolar organizer region (NOR) of the nucleus is suitable for prognostic assessments, is known by the acronym of argyrophilic nucleolar organizer region (AgNOR) (Boldy, 1989). Nucleolin, an RNA-binding acidic protein present in the nucleolus, functions in ribosomal transcription reactions and binds silver molecules with high affinity Acidic proteins such as nucleolin are the NOR-associated proteins (NORAPs) (Colecchia and Leopardi, 1992). The diagnostic possibilities inherent in AgNORs first attracted attention 15 years ago. Numerous experiments have shown that the number of AgNORs is significantly higher in malignant tumors than in physiologic, reactive, or benign processes. It has been demonstrated that the number of AgNORs per nucleus can be regarded as one of the hallmarks of proliferation and that mean AgNOR counts are good indicators of the degree of malignancy (Vajdovich, et al. 2004).

. Crystal violet is a basic dye which has a high affinity for the highly acidic chromatin of mitotic cells. Mitotic cells are stained magenta and stand out distinctly against a light blue background of resting cells. As many studies show that The significantly increased mitotic counts with 1% crystal violet suggests that this stain provides a crisp staining facilitating the identification of mitotic figures even at a lower magnification as compared to an H/E-stained section. (Ankle and Kale, 2007).

Justification

Thirty percent to 80% of the malignancies of the oral cavity arise from premalignant lesions, such as leukoplakia, erythroplakia, and oral submucous fibrosis, so we to determine simple, cost-effective, slective and specific cytological technique that assess cellular proliferative activity among Toombak dippers. Now days, Toombak dipping became a prevalence tradition not only in Nile Province, but all Sudan states. So, this study was carried out to confirm these data by using other specific methods that will help in establishing oral screening program in the Sudan.

CHAPTER TWO

Review of Literature

2.1 Anatomy and Histology:

The oral cavity is the first portion of the alimentary canal , which includes the front two-third of the tongue, the upper and lower gums (the gingiva); the lining inside the cheeks and lips is the buccal and labial mucosa. The mouth floor under the tongue and the bony top of the mouth is the hard palate. The small area behind the wisdom teeth (the retromolar trigone).The entire oral cavity is lined by stratified squamous epithelium, which varies in thickness and Keratinization according to anatomic and functional sites. The degree of normal surface Keratinization (genetically predetermined) varies. The hard palate, gingiva and dorsal of the tongue are Keratinized. Oropharynxes, soft palate, lateral and ventral tongue and floor of mouth are non-keratinized. The buccal and labial mucosa is intermediate between these two extremes (Burkitt, et al. 1996). Normal squamous epithelium of the oral shed cells resembling superficial and intermediate squamous cells of the vagina and cervix, except that, nuclear Pyknosis is not observed. Such cells either occur singly or in clusters and are identical with squamous cells that are found in specimens of sputum and of saliva. Fully keratinized squamous cells without visible nuclei are a common component of oral smears, especially from the palate, and do not necessarily reflect a significant abnormality. All stages of transition between non keratinized and keratinized cells may be observed. Other cells like Smaller Parabasal cells may be observed if the surface of the epithelium is vigorously scraped, or if an epithelial defect, such as ulceration is present. Mucus-producing columnar cells originated in the nasopharynx or in the salivary glands ducts may occasionally be observed. A vigorous scrape of tonsillar area or the base of tongue may result in shedding of the lymphocytes, singly or in clusters (Koss, 2005).

2.2 Oral flora:

Oral flora, especially in patients with poor oral hygiene, is rich in a variety of saprophytic fungi and bacteria. A protozoon, Entamoeba gingivalis, is fairly common. The presence of these organisms does not necessarily indicate an inflammatory process in the oral cavity (Koss, 2005).

2.3 Inflammatory Disorders:

2.3.1 Acute and Chronic Inflammatory Processes:

Superficial erosion or ulceration of the squamous epithelium occurs frequently in the course of diffuse or localized inflammatory processes or poor oral hygiene. As a result, the normal population of superficial and intermediate squamous cells in smears is partially or completely replaced by parabasal squamous cells from the deeper epithelial layers. Such cells may be varying in shape and size. In the presence of diffuse stomatitis or gingivitis, the preponderance of the irregularly shaped parabasal cells may result in an initial impression of a significant epithelial abnormality. Close attention to nuclear detail will prevent erroneous diagnosis of cancer. In chronic ulcerative processes, mono- and multi-nucleated macrophages may also occur. Purulent exudate or leukocytes of various types are a common component of smears in these situations. Plasma cells are frequently observed, particularly in smears from the posterior oral cavity or pharynx (Koss, 2005).

2.3.2 Specific inflammatory Conditions:

Actinomycosis: Actinomyces species are common saprophytes of the oral cavity. Usually found within tonsillar crypts, and are usually of no clinical significance. However, they may invade the traumatized or ulcerated mucosa and form abscess.

Oral herpes: this common disorder characterized by blisters and painful ulceration, is caused by herpes virus type 1 that is usually responsible for inflammatory lesions. Herpes virus type 1 can be identified by the characteristic nuclear changes.

Moniliasis (Thrush): Clinically, moniliasis forms a characteristic white coating of the oral cavity. This organism may be identified by finding the characteristic fungal spores and pseudohyphae. This harmless infection, previously occurring mainly in debilitated patients and diabetics, has been recognized as one of the first manifestations of the acquired immunodeficiency syndrome (AIDS).

Blastomycosis: paracoccidiomycosis (South American blastomycosis), is a common and serious disorder in Latin American countries. Detected by presence of its yeast.

Candidiasis: is common in infants, but in adults it may signify immune deficiency or other illness. Oral candidiasis may present as pseudomembranous candidiasis, glossitis, or perleche (angular cheilitis).

Human Papilloma Virus (HPV): HPV now has been documented in benign and malignant lesion of the oral cavity. HPV types 2,4,6,11,13 and 32 observed in benign lesions, including leukoplakia, and HPV types 16 and 18 in oral carcinomas (takahashi, et al. 1998).

2.4 Benign Oral lesions:

Changes in oral squamous cells in deficiency diseases: in diseases associated with deficiencies in vitamin B12 and folic acid,such as pernicious anemia,the squamous cells of the oral mucosa may show significant enlargement of both the nucleus and cytoplasm (boen,1957).

2.4.1 Other benign disorders:

These include the benign leukoplakia in which heavy keratin formation on the surface of oral epithelium is a common phenomenon and hairy oral leukoplakia in AIDS patients. Darier white's disease (keratosis follicularis); in which the disease characterized by disturbance of keratinization. white sponge nevus of canon that characterized by spongy hypertrophy of squamous epithelium of the oral cavity. Hereditary benign intraepithelial dyskeratosis (Witkop) in this rare hereditary disorder, there is formation of white spongy folds and plaques of thickened mucosa within the oral cavity. Other rare benign disorder pemphigus vulgaris the disease that caused by antibodies to desmoglein 3 and changes in oral epthilial cells caused by radiation therapy and chemotherapy (koss, 2005).

2.5 Premalignant Oral Lesions:

Leukoplakia and erythroplakia are two clinical lesions widely considered to be premalignant. However, using clinical features to classify lesions is difficult because they vary in appearance and are likely to be interpreted subjectively by the clinician. A histopathologic diagnosis is generally more indicative of premalignant change than clinically apparent alterations. The term leukoplakia is sometimes used inappropriately to indicate a premalignant condition. In fact, the term describes a white plaque that does not rub off and cannot be clinically identified as another entity. Most cases of leukoplakia are a hyperkeratotic response to an irritant and are asymptomatic, but about 20% of leukoplakic lesions show evidence of dysplasia or carcinoma at first clinical

14

recognition (Axell, et al. 1996). The term erythroleukoplakia has been used to describe leukoplakias with a red component. An erythroplakia is a red lesion that cannot be classified as another entity. Far less common than leukoplakia, erythroplakia has a much greater probability (91%) of showing signs of dysplasia or malignancy at the time of diagnosis (Shafer, et al. 1975).

2.6 Oral Cancer:

Oral cancer is part of the group of head and neck cancers. Oral cancer can develop in any part of the oral cavity or oropharynx. Most oral cancers begin in the tongue and in the floor of the mouth. Almost all oral cancers begin in the squemous cells that cover the surfaces of the oral. Therefore, classified as squamous cell carcinomas more than 90% of the time. According to the degree of differentiation, three subtypes are defined: (1) well-differentiated squamous cell carcinoma showing more than 75% keratinization; (2) moderately differentiated squamous cell carcinoma with 25-75% keratinization; and (3) poorly differentiated squamous cell carcinoma with less than 25% keratinization. The majority of cases are of moderate differentiation (Zarbo, 1988). Other rare variants of oral, head and neck carcinomas include pseudoglandular, basaloid and small cell neuroendocrine carcinomas. The latter two being radiosensitive. Because these tumors share histologic features with other neoplasms (i.e., melanomas, neuroblastomas, lymphomas), the use of specific immunohistochemical markers is warranted (Million, et al. 1994).

2.6.1 Epidemiology of oral Cancer:

Worldwide, more than 500,000 new cases of oral cancer are diagnosed each year (Stewart, et al. 2008). In 2008, there were 22,900 cases of oral cavity cancer, 12,250 cases of laryngeal cancer, and 12,410 cases of pharyngeal cancer in the United States.

Seventy-four hundred Americans are projected to die of these cancers (ridge, et al. 2008). The number of new cases of head and neck cancers in the United States was 40,490 in 2006, accounting for about 3% of adult malignancies and 11,170 patients died of their disease in 2006 (jemal, et al. 2006). Squamous cell carcinoma, which arises from the oral mucosal lining, accounts for over 90 percent of these tumors. Mortality rates show similar differentials: 4.5 per 100,000 per year for males, 1.7 per 100,000 per year for females. This gender difference is also evident in the lifetime risks of developing oral cancer: 1.5% for males and 0.7% for females (Brad, et al. 2002). Oral cancer is a disease of increasing age: approximately 95% of cases occur in people older than 40 years; with an average age at diagnosis of approximately 60 years.the age related incidence suggests that time-dependent factors result in the initiation and promotion of genetic events that result in malignant change (Mashburg, 1989). Five-Years relative survival rates Based on data from 1983-1990, the overall 5-year survival rate for oral cancer was 52.5%. Females fared somewhat better than males (58% versus 50%). Blacks did far worse than whites; only 34% of blacks survived 5 years after the initial diagnosis, compared with 55% of whites. There was a great difference within the black subgroup; however, as the survival rate for black males was only 28%, versus 47% for black females (Gloeckler, et al. 1994).

2.6.2 Etiology of Oral Cancer:

Evidence of the etiologic factors of squamous cell carcinoma is based on studies of at-risk groups, differences in incidence of disease, laboratory studies of malignant tissues, and animal studies. The incidence of oral cancer is clearly age related, which may reflect declining immune surveillance with age, time for the accumulation of genetic changes, and duration of exposure to initiators and promoters (these include chemical and physical irritants, viruses, hormonal effects, cellular aging, and decreased immunologic surveillance). Tobacco and alcohol are acknowledged risk factors for oral and oropharyngeal cancer (Feldman, et al. 1975). Consideration of risk factors should recognize that many molecular events governing control of cell cycles are influenced by viruses. Those most commonly implicated in oral cancer transformation have been the human papilloma virus (HPV), herpes group viruses, and the adenoviruses. Of these, HPV and herpes have been the most thoroughly studied and are now considered to be the most likely "synergistic viruses" involved in human oral cancer. The herpes viruses most often linked to oral cancer are the Epstein-Barr virus (EBV) and cytomegalovirus (CMV); both EBV (DNA) and CMV. In HPV, The genotypes most often found in oral carcinoma are HPV 16 and 18, but HPV can also be found in normal oral mucosa (Greer, et al. 1990).

Tobacco was first introduced in Europe by Spanish and Portuguese explorers of America in the early 16th century. The different ways in which tobacco is used lead to considerable variation in appearance, site and frequency of the lesions associated with the tobacco habit. In western countries, cigarettes, cigars and pipes are the major ways in which tobacco is used, but chewing tobacco and snuff dipping (smokeless tobacco) have become more popular in recent years. Tobacco contains potent carcinogens, including nitrosamines (nicotine), polycyclic aromatic hydrocarbons, nitrosodicthanolamine, nitrosoproline, and polonium. Nicotine is a powerful and addicting drug (Graham, et al. 1977).

Smokeless tobacco also contains carcinogens, some at extremely high levels. It is especially significant that the preparation of smokeless tobacco products, which entails curing, fermentation, and aging, occurs under conditions favouring the formation of tobacco-specific N-nitrosamines (TSNAs) from nicotine and other tobacco alkaloids such as nornicotine, anatabine, and anabasine. During tobacco chewing and snuff dipping, it is likely that additional amounts of carcinogenic TSNAs are also formed endogenously in the oral cavity.

Two of the six TSNAs identified in smokeless tobacco, N'-nitrosonornicotine (NNN) and 4(methylnitrosamino)-1 3-pyridyl-1-butanone (NNK), are strong carcinogens in mice, rats, and hamsters, capable of inducing both benign and malignant tumors of the oral and nasal cavity as well as of the lung, esophagus, and pancreas. Polynuclear aromatic hydrocarbons (PAHs) in tobacco smoke have been implicated extensively in oral carcinogenesis, and NNK and NNN, which are found in both tobacco and tobacco smoke, likely play a major etiological role in cancers of the oral cavity (Hoffman, et al.1995).

2.6.2.1 Toombak:

In the Sudan, snuff, locally known as toombak, was introduced approximately 400 years ago. It is always processed into a loose moist form and its use is widespread in the country. Tobacco used for manufacture of the toombak is of the species Nicotiana rustica and the fermented ground powder is mixed with an aqueous solution of sodium bicarbonate. The resultant product is moist, with a strong aroma, highly addictive and its use is widespread particularly among males. Its pH range is 8-11, moisture content ranges 6-60% and nicotine content is from 8 to 102 mg/g dry wt and tobacco specific nitrosamines TSNAs contents in micrograms (N'-nitrosonornicotine NNN 420-1 550; 4-(methyl-nitrosamino)-l-(3- pyridyl)-l- butanone NNK 620-7 870; N'-nitrosoanatabine NAT 20-290).

Toombak dippers develop a clinically and histologically characteristic lesion at the site of dipping. The risk for cancer of the oral cavity among toombak users was high (RR 7.3-73.0-fold). The use of toombak plays a significant role in etiology of oral squamous cell carcinoma (OSCCs), with the tobacco specific nitrosamines present in toombak possibly acting as principal carcinogens (Ahmed and Mahgoob, 2007).

A retrospective study involving 78 cases of oral carcinoma was conducted to investigate their association with the habit of taking 'snuff-dipping'. It was found that 50 (81%) of the 62 questioned patients used snuff in the form of saffa. It was also found that carcinomatous changes usually developed in the area of the mouth where the snuff was habitually placed. It was concluded that the association between saffa and development of oral carcinoma is likely to be causal (Elbeshir, et al.1998).

2.6.2.2 Toombak and Oral Cancer in Sudan:

Survey data on the prevalence of use of oral snuff (Toombak) and cigarette consumption according to various demographic factors are needed in the Sudan. A house to house cross-sectional survey of a random population sample of 4,535 households was performed. Of the 23,367 household members identified, 21,648 (92.6%) eligible individuals were questioned about tobacco use. Among children and adolescents (4–17 years) prevalence of tobacco use was quite low (2%, range 1–2%), but there was an abrupt increase up to 25% in late adolescence. Among the adult population aged 18 years and older the prevalences of toombak use (34%) and cigarette smoking (12%) among males were significantly higher than among females (2.5 and 0.9%, respectively). The prevalence of toombak use among the male population aged 18 years and older was significantly higher in the rural than in the urban areas (35% vs 24%), while cigarette smoking had a higher prevalence in urban areas (18% vs 12%). The highest rates of toombak use were found in rural areas among the male population ages 30 years and older (mean 46.6%, range 45–47%). So, in view of the high prevalence of tobacco use, especially of toombak, among the population surveyed, there is an urgent need to educate the public on the health consequences of these habits (Idris, et al. 1998).

Data from 1,916 cases of oral neoplasm occurring in the Sudan in a 16-years period, from January 1970 to December 1985, were retrieved and analyzed. The study revealed a relatively high frequency of oral neoplasm in comparing with neighboring countries. Squamous cell carcinoma was the most common oral malignancy (66.5%), followed by tumors of the salivary gland (14.7%), neoplasms of nonodontogenic and non-epithelial origin (9.6%) and odontogenic neoplasms (8.6%). Men had a higher frequency than women. The older age group of both genders showed a relatively high frequency of Squamous cell carcinoma. Among northern Sudanese there was a high frequency of squamous cell carcinoma, while southern Sudanese showed a high rate of odontogenic and salivary gland neoplasm's. The use of Toombak has been stated to play a major role in the etiology of oral squamous cell carcinoma in the Sudan, and is suspected to be with neoplasm of the salivary glands. Therefore, Oral cancer (OC) mortality in the Sudan is very high, particularly among men due to the habit of Toombak use (tobacco specific nitroseamine (TSN) rich tobacco) (Idris, et al. 1995).

Clinical (n = 281) and histopathological (n = 141) characteristics of Toombak-associated oral mucosal lesions detected in an epidemiological study in northern Sudan in 1992/93 are described. The lesional site in the majority of Toombak users was the anterior lower labial groove and the lower labial mucosa. Four degrees (1-4) of clinical severity of lesions, similar to those used to characterise Swedish snuff-dipper's lesions were applied. An association between the severity of mucosal lesions and longer lifetime duration (> 10 years) of toombak use was found, but the severity was not related to the daily frequency of the habit. Parakeratosis, pale surface staining of the epithelium and basal cell hyperplasia were commonly observed, but epithelial dysplasia was infrequent (10/141). The most significant observation was a PAS-positive amorphous deposit between the lamina propria and the submucosa, found in 25/141 biopsies. The clinical and histopathological features of Toombak lesions are closely similar to Swedish moist snuff-dipper's lesions and this may reflect the high alkalinity of these products, resulting in an alkaline burn on the oral mucosa following chronic exposure. The low prevalence of epithelial dysplasia implies a low risk of malignant transformation. Nevertheless, the high concentrations of tobacco-specific nitrosamines present in Toombak, and the high prevalence of oral cancer in Sudan, mandate biopsy and careful histopathological analysis of any such lesions detected in habitual users (Idris, et al.1996).

2.6.3 Diagnosis:
2.6.3.1 Clinical Diagnosis:
Common symptoms of oral cancer include: Patches inside the oral and lips that are white (leukoplakia), a mixture of red and white (erythroleukoplakia), or red (erythroplakia), bleeding in the oral, loose teeth, difficulty or pain when swallowing and an earache. The clinician or dentist checks the oral and throat for red or white patches, lumps, swelling, or other abnormalities. This exam includes looking carefully at the soft and hard palates of the oral, back of the throat, insides of the cheeks and lips, Sides of the tongue and near lymph nodes(Murata, et al. 1996). Listening is an important part of

this examination. The sound of one's voice and speech are important in consideration of the location of tumors as a "hot potato" voice may signal the presence of an oropharyngeal tumor whereas a raspy, hoarse voice could be the first sign of a laryngeal neoplasm. Throughout this oral, head and neck cancers examination, it is helpful to remember to look, listen, and feel every site that is being examined (Mashberg and Samit, 1995).

2.6.3.2 Vital tissue staining:

Tolonium chloride, more commonly referred to as Tolidine Blue, has been used for more than 40 years to aid in detection of mucosal abnormalities of the cervix and the oral cavity. Tolidine Blue is a metachromatic vital dye that may bind preferentially to tissues undergoing rapid cell division (such as inflammatory, regenerative and neoplastic tissue), to sites of DNA change associated with oral potentially malignant lesions or both. The binding results in the staining of abnormal tissue in contrast to adjacent normal mucosa. A prior meta-analysis summarized 12 studies conducted between 1964 and 1984 and reported an overall sensitivity of 93.5 percent and specificity of 73.3 percent (Patton, et al. 2008).

2.6.3.3 Visualization adjuncts:

Several visualization adjuncts, described below, are intended for use as adjuncts to the standard visual and tactile oral examination under incidence light. They function under the assumption that mucosal tissues undergoing abnormal metabolic or structural changes have different absorbance and reflectance profiles when exposed to various forms of light or energy. Described as a chemiluminescent light detection system, was developed from predicate devices to detect cervical neoplasia. After receiving application of acetic acid, sites of epithelial proliferation, having cells with altered nuclear structure, are purported to preferentially reflect the low energy blue-white light emitted by a device generating an "acetowhite" change. The proposed mechanism of tissue fluorescence is that mucosal tissues have a reflective and absorptive pattern based on naturally occurring fluorophores in the tissue. Tissue fluorescence in the oral cavity is variable and is affected by structural changes, metabolic activity, the presence of hemoglobin in the tissue, vessel dilatation and, possibly, inflammation. This variability has not been defined. Exposure to blue light spectra (400-460 nanometers) may maximize a differential profile in areas undergoing neoplastic change in which a loss of fluorescence visualization is reported (Patton, et al. 2008).

2.6.3.4 Biopsy:

The gold standard diagnostic test for oral mucosal lesions that is suggestive of premalignancy or malignancy remains tissue biopsy with histopathological examination (Patton, et al. 2008). Even though the biopsy study is fundamental, it is an invasive technique with surgical implications, technique limitations for professionals and psychological implications for most patients. Also it presents limitations when the lesions are large and in these cases it is important to select the most appropriate site of biopsy.in addition to the diagnostic method with limited sensitivity where one of the most important features is the subjective interpretation of the examining pathologist (Spafford, et al. 2001).

2.6.3.5 Application of cytology in diagnosing premalignant or malignant oral lesions:

Exfoliative cytology is a diagnosis complementary exam, based on the observation of cells that are constantly exfoliating from the epithelium, as a consequence of this tissue's natural maturation process. Early detection of a premalignant or cancerous oral

23

lesion promises to improve the survival and the morbidity of patients suffering from these conditions. Cytological study of oral cells is a non-aggressive technique that is well accepted by the patient, and is therefore an attractive option for the early diagnosis of oral cancer, including epithelial atypia and squamous cell carcinoma. In recent decades, there are dramatic switch from histopathological to molecular methods of disease diagnosis and exfoliative cytology has gained importance as a rapid and simple method for screening and diagnosis oral diseases. So Identification of high-risk oral premalignant lesions and intervention at premalignant stages could constitute one of the keys to reducing the mortality, morbidity and cost of treatment associated with oral squamous cell carcinoma (Epstein, et al. 2002).

2.6.3.5.1 Cytological Studies in the Sudan:

Prevalence of oral cancer is high in Sudan and the disease is attributed to N-nitrosamine rich oral snuff consumption. A screening procedure for oral cancer and precancers, Exfoliative cytology (EFC) was applied to a retrospective cohort to assess the presence and severity of oral epithelial atypia (ET) in 300 subjects (100 toombak dippers; 100 cigarette smokers; 100 non-tobacco users) without prior knowledge of the subjects' tobacco exposure. Five patients with oral squamous cell carcinoma (OSCC) were included as internal controls. ET was ascertained in 29 subjects and could not be ascertained in the remaining 271. Among the 29 subjects with ET, there were 11 (38%) toombak dippers, 14 (48%) cigarette smokers and 4 (14%) non-tobacco users. Among the 271 subjects without ET, there were 89 (33%) toombak dippers, 86 (32%) cigarette smokers and 96 (35%) non-tobacco users. ET was found in all the 5 control cases with OSCC. For the ET among toombak dippers and cigarette smokers, adjusted OR and the 95% CI were found to be 3 (0.91-9.7) and 4 (1.2-12.3), respectively. In view of these findings, the use of exfoliative cytology for detection and assessment of oral epithelial atypia was proposed (Ahmed, et al. 2003).

To investigate the possible causal association between squamous-cell carcinomas of the oral cavity and use of Toombak, the history of use of this substance was retrospectively compared in 375 patients with squamous-cell carcinomas of the lip, buccal cavity and floor of mouth. And 271 patients diagnosed squamous carcinomas of the tongue, palate and maxillary sinus. Compared with 204 patients exhibiting non-squamous oral and non-oral malignant neoplasms and 2,820 individuals who had no malignancy were selected from the general population. The study revealed that the high prevalence of oral cancer in the Sudan is largely due to chronic use of Toombak. The adjusted ORs associated with toombak dipping for the first case group, cancer of the lip, buccal cavity and floor of mouth in comparison with the hospital and population control groups, were 7.3 and 3.9 (95% confidence limits, 4.3-12.4 and 2.9-5.3) respectively and among long-term users the adjusted ORs were 11.0 and 4.3 (95% confidence limits, 4.8-25.1 and 2.9-6.3) respectively. The elevated risk found when investigating intra-oral cancers of sites in direct contact with toombak quid compared to those with little or no contact, confirms the hypothesis that direct contact with tissues is an important factor in tobacco carcinogenesis in the mouth. The increased risk associated with the use of toombak is of particular concern in view of its wide consumption in the Sudan (Idris, et al.1994).

2.6.3.5.2 Argyrophilic nuclear organizer regions (AgNOR):

Nucleolar organiser regions (NORs) are DNA sequences on the short arms of acrocentric chromosomes, which encode ribosomal RNA. Owing to their argyrophilic nucleoproteins, silver stained NORs (AgNORs) can be visualised in routine histological or cytological preparations as black or dark brown dots in the interphase nucleus. AgNOR frequency is considered to be an index of transcriptional activity and hence a measure of the cellular mitotic potential. The mean number of AgNORs in each nucleus (AgNOR count) is now widely used in tumour pathology as a diagnostic and prognostic marker, because it can discriminate between malignant and benign or reactive proliferations, and has been shown to correlate well with the degree of aggressiveness and patient survival in many different cancers, including haematological malignancies(Mamaev, et al.1997). The silver stain was originally used to demonstrate the NORs of chromosomes, to evaluate their function, and to identify chromosomes in cytogenetic preparations. The technique was simplified and was first applied to histological sections by Ploton, et al. (1986). It was subsequently popularized, especially by Crocker (1990) and the staining protocol that Crocker described has been used by most workers in the field. It suffers from limited reliability, background staining, precipitates, and fading of the sections. Factors were identified that affect these problems. The oxidation-reduction level and gelatin used are particularly important. An improved procedure is presented which incorporates pre- reduction of the sections, selection of an optimal gelatin, and post- treatment of the sections to produce a permanent preparation. It is compatible with many fixatives and with other stains used before or after the silver stain (Luther and Lindner, 1993).

The diagnostic accuracy of AgNOR-analysis as an adjunctive diagnostic tool of conventional oral exfoliative cytology taken from suspicious lesions was assessed. Cytological diagnosis obtained from brush biopsies of macroscopically suspicious lesions of the oral mucosa from 75 patients (final diagnoses: 53 histologically proven squamous cell carcinomas, 11 leukoplakias and other inflammatory oral lesions) and from 11 patients with normal mucosa as a negative control group were compared with histological and/or clinical follow-ups. Five smears were doubtful and seven suspicious for tumor cells in the cytologic report. Number of AgNOR's was counted in 100 squamous epithelial cell-nuclei per slide after silver-staining. Sensitivity of the cytological diagnosis alone on oral smears for the detection of squamous carcinomas was 92.5%, specificity 100%, positive predictive value was 100% and negative 84.6%. The best cut-off value of the mean number of AgNOR dots per nucleus distinguishing benign from malignant cells was 4.8. The percentage of nuclei with more than three AgNORs had a cut-off level of 70%. Applying these methods to twelve doubtful or suspicious cytological diagnoses was able to correctly establish the diagnosis of malignancy in ten cases of histologically proven cancers and to reveal benignity in two histologically proven cases. Smears from brushings of visible oral lesions, if clinically considered as suspicious for cancer, are an easily practicable, non-invasive, painless, safe and accurate screening method for detection of oral cancerous lesions. AgNOR-analysis may be a useful adjunct to other methods in routine cytological diagnosis of oral cancer that can help to solve cytology suspicious or doubtful cases (Torsten, et al. 2003).

In study aimed to assess cellular proliferative activity of clinically healthy oral mucosal epithelial cells of Toombak dippers and smokers by means of AgNOR counts and nuclear areas via nuclear morphometry. Smears were collected from normal-appearing mouth floor mucosa and tongue of 75 toombak dippers, 75 smokers and 50 non-tobacco users between the ages of 20 and 70 with a mean age of 36 years. AgNORs were counted in the first 50 well-fixed, nucleated squamous cells and nuclear areas were calculated via microscopic stage micrometer. Cytological atypia was ascertained in 6 tobacco users and could not be ascertained in non-tobacco users. Statistically mean AgNOR numbers per nucleus in the non-tobacco users (2.45 ± 0.30) was lower than the toombak dippers (3.081 ± 0.39, $p<0.004$), and the smokers (2.715 ± 0.39, $p<0.02$), and mean nuclear areas of epithelial cells of toombak dippers (6.081 ± 0.39, $p<0.009$) and smokers (5.68 ± 10.08, $p<0.01$) was also significantly higher than non-smokers (5.39 ± 9.4). The mean number of nuclei having more than 3 AgNORs was 28%, 19% and 7% in toombak dippers, smokers and non-tobacco users, respectively. These findings support the view that toombak dipping and smoking are severe risk factors for oral mucosal proliferative lesions and exfoliative cytology is valid for screening of oral mucosal lesions (Ahmed and babiker, 2009).

2.6.3.5.3 Buccal cell micronuclei (MNs):

The buccal cell micronucleus (MN) is defined as a microscopically visible, round or oval cytoplasmic chromatin mass next to the nucleus. Micronuclei originate from aberrant mitosis and consist of acentric chromosomes, chromatid fragments or whole chromosomes that have failed to be incorporated in the daughter nuclei during mitosis. The micronuclei test is the most frequent technique used to detect chromosome breakage or mitotic interference thought to be associated with increased risk for cancer (Stich, et al. 1982). The frequency of micronucleated cell was measured to assess genotoxic damage in tobacco products users. When compared to other body sites, the mouth offers a unique opportunity to define biomarkers because the mouth permits non-invasive examination in longitudinal studies of smoking and smokeless tobacco-associated acute and chronic diseases. As micronuclei are derived from chromosomal fragments and whole chromosomes lagging behind in anaphase, the micronuclei assay can be used to show both clastogenic and aneugenic effects. Micronuclei formation is undoubtedly an important mechanism associated with chromosome loss (Hazare, et al.1998).

Earlier studies have shown that false-positive results in the micronucleus (MN) frequency can be obtained as a result of using Romanowsky-type stains such as Giemsa, May-Grunwald Giemsa and/or Leishmann's, which leads to inaccurate assessment of DNA damage. In a study investigating MN frequency in relation to the staining techniques in the buccal mucosa(BM) of smokers against non-smokers, a 4- to 5-fold increase in MN frequency in smokers was found using Romanowsky stains, which are not DNA-specific. However, when a specific DNA fluorescent dye (e.g., 4, 6-diamidino-2- phenylindole (DAPI), Feulgen or Acridine orange) was used there were no significant differences between these groups. Romanowsky stains have been shown to increase the number of false positives as they positively stain keratin bodies that are often mistaken for micronuclei and are therefore not appropriate for this type of analysis. For these reasons, it is advisable to avoid Romanowsky stains in favor of DNA-specific fluorescent-based stains such as propidium iodide, DAPI, Feulgen, Hoechst 33258 or Acridine Orange42. It is recommended that Feulgen be used because permanent slides can be obtained that can be viewed under both transmitted and/or fluorescent light conditions (Nersesyan, et al. 2006). Criteria for identifying cells with micronuclei are characterized by the presence of both a main nucleus and one or more smaller nuclear structures called micronuclei (MNi). The micronuclei are round or oval in shape and their diameter should range between 1/3 and 1/16 of the main nucleus. MNi have the same staining intensity and texture as the main nucleus. The MNi must be located within the cytoplasm **of** the cells. Most cells with MNi will contain only one MN but it is possible to find cells with two or more MNi. Cells withmultipleMNi are rare in healthy subjects but become more common in individuals exposed to radiation or other genotoxic agents(Tolbert, et al. 1992). Baseline frequencies for micronucleated cells in the BM are usually within the 0.5–2.5MNi/1,000 cells range (Holland, et al. 2008).

In a study aimed to evaluate the micronuclei (MN) in buccal mucosa of healthy individuals from southern India, Who were regularly chewing a mixture of betel leaf, areca nut and tobacco. A total of 44 subjects were examined. The study population included 15 chewers, 14 chewers with smoking habit and 15 controls with the mean age of 38.57 ± 0.54, 34.50 ± 0.95, and 33.28 ± 0.89 years, respectively. The mean percentage of MN was 1.90 ± 1.03 in chewers, 2.00 ± 1.12 in chewers with smoking habits and 0.81 ± 0.66 in controls. There was no significant difference between the mean percentages of the two experimental groups. It can be concluded that a mixture of betel leaf, areca nut, and tobacco is unsafe for oral health (Sellappa, et al. 2009).

In a study of 120 healthy subjects, the frequency of micronuclei of oral epithelial cells was three times greater in smokers (n = 50) than nonsmokers (n = 70); recorded micronuclei frequency values were 1.50 ± 0.47% and 0.55 ± 0.32%, respectively ($P <$ 0.05). Neither age nor gender correlated with the level of micronuclei (Konopacka, et al.2003). In a study the evaluation of micronuclei in buccal mucosa cells of habitual Maras Powder users (smokeless tobacco). There was no difference in the micronuclei of buccal cells of subjects who smoked or chewed smokeless tobacco (maras powder).

Buccal cells of both groups showed a higher frequency of micronuclei than nonusers (nonsmokers, nonchewers) (Ozkul, et al. 1997).

2.6.3.5.4 Selective cytochemical staining of mitotic figures using1% crystal violet stain:

Mitosis of cells gives rise to tissue integrity. Defects during mitosis bring about abnormalities. Excessive proliferation of cells due to increased mitosis is one such outcome, which is the hallmark in precancer and cancer. The localization of proliferating cells or their precursors may not be obvious and easy. Establishing an easy way to distinguish these mitotic cells will help in grading and understanding their biological potential. Although, immunohistochemistry is an advanced method in use, the cost and time factor makes it less feasible for many laboratories. Selective histochemical stains like toluidine blue, giemsa and crystal violet have been used in tissues including the developing brain, neural tissue and skin. The distinction between a pyknotic nucleus, an apoptotic cell and a mitotic cell in a routinely stained tissue section may pose a problem. Errors in identifying a mitotic cell can thus weaken the reliability of histological or cytological grading due to the loose use of morphologic criteria. Combination of stains and modification of the existing histochemical techniques can overcome these problems. A literature search revealed numerous selective stains like crystal violet, toluidine blue and giemsa which highlight chromatin patterns. These stains have been used in brain tissue, uterus and breast carcinoma. Crystal violet is a basic dye which has a high affinity for the highly acidic chromatin of mitotic cells. Mitotic cells are stained magenta and stand out distinctly against a light blue background of resting cells. As many studies show that the significantly increased mitotic counts with 1% crystal violet suggests that this stain provides a crisp staining facilitating the identification of mitotic figures even at a lower magnification as compared to an H/E-stained section. Criteria to identify the mitotic cells: the nuclear membrane must be absent indicating that cells have passed the prophase, clear, hairy extensions of nuclear material (condensed chromosomes) must be present-either clotted (beginning metaphase), in a plane (metaphase / anaphase) or in separate clots (telophase) and two parallel, clearly separate chromosome clots to be counted as if they are separate (Ankle and Kale, 2007).

In a study aimed to compare the staining of mitotic cells in haematoxylin and eosin with that in crystal violet and to compare the number of mitotic figures present in normal oral mucosa, epithelial dysplasia and oral squamous cell carcinoma in crystal violet-stained sections with that in H and E-stained sections. No mitotic cells were seen either in the crystal violet-stained or in the H and E-stained sections in ten cases of normal oral mucosa. A statistically significant increase in the mean mitotic count was observed in crystal violet-stained sections of epithelial dysplasia as compared to the H and E-stained sections (p = 0.0327). A similar increase in the mitotic counts was noted in crystal violet-stained sections of oral squamous cell carcinoma as compared to the H and E-stained sections(p = 0.0443). One per cent crystal violet provides a definite advantage over the H and E-stained sections in selectively staining the mitotic figures (Ankle and Kale, 2007).

CHAPTER THREE

Objectives

Objectives:

To compare the cytological methods used in the assessment of cellular proliferative activity agnor, micronucleus assay, crystal violet (selective mitotic figure stain) and papanicolaou stain applied to oral epithelium of Toombak dippers.

CHAPTER FOUR

Materials and methods

Study design:

This is a retrospective case control cohort study, carried out among Toombak users.

Study Population:

A total 0f 210 participants were examined in this study of which two hundred apparently healthy individuals: one hundred were Toombak users (ascertained as cases) the remaining hundred were non-tobacco users (ascertained as controls). And ten were patients with Oral Squamous Cell Carcinoma (OSCC), as an internal control.

Sample Size: is calculated according to the Formula:

$$n= \frac{t^2 \times p(1-p)}{m}$$

Description:

n=required sample size

t = confidence level at 95% (standard value of 1.96)

p = estimated prevalence.

m = margin of error at 5% (standard value of 0.05)

Ethical Consideration:

Each participant was asked to sign an ethical consent form before taking of the specimen and filling of the questioner.

Samples collection and smears preparation:

Four smears were made from each specimen using a flat sterile wooden tongue depressor. The surface epithelium of buccal mucosa was scraped mainly the dip site and the materials were prepared in clean grease free frosted glass slides. All smears were fixed immediately by conventional fixative for Pap smears (95% ethyl alcohol) while they were wet for 15 minutes.

Papanicolaou Procedure:

-Fix slides in 95% ethyl alcohol fixative for 15 minutes.

-70% alcohol 2 minutes.

- 50% alcohol 2 minutes.

- Tap water 2 minutes.

- Stain in Harris Haematoxylin 2 minutes.

- Rinse in tap water briefly.

- Differentiate in 1% acid alcohol 5 seconds.

- Blue in tap water for 10 minutes.

- Dehydrate to 95% ethyl alcohol.

- Stain in orange G 2 minutes.

- Rinse in 95% ethyl alcohol.

- Stain in Eosin Azure 50 2 minutes.

- Wash in 95% ethyl alcohol.

- Rinse in absolute alcohol 2 minutes.

- Clear in xylene.

- Mount sections in DPX (Bancroft, et al. 2002).

Cytological Interpretation:

The presence of two or more of the following features indicated the presence of epithelial atypia: nuclear enlargement associated with increased nuclear cytoptasmic ratio, hyperchromatism, chromatin clumping with moderately prominent nucleolation , irregular nuclear borders, bi or multinuclation, increased keratinisation, scantiness of the cytoplasm and variations in size and or shape of the cells and nuclei. For each of these features, three possible grades were provided. The first grade allows for the fact that the characteristic may be completely absent (i.e. "none") or present in its normal form (i.e. "normal"). The other two grades (slight or marked) allow for different degrees of severity (mild, moderate or severe). The examiner had been trained in the calibration of the scoring by screening of normal and abnormal cytological smears in comparison with an atlas containing various abnormalities of the different characteristics (Ahmed, et al. 2003).

Silver nitrate:

Fifty present silver nitrates, 2% gelatine in 1% formic acid were the component. smears were hydrated in 70% alcohol for 2 minutes and rinsed in distilled water then incubated in freshly prepared working solution (2:1) for 45 minutes at dark and moist area, then washed by distil water, 5% sodium thiosulphate and dehydrated in two changes of absolute alcohol, cleared in two changes of Xylene and mounted with DPX medium.

Result interpretation:

All quality control measures were adopted during specimen collection and processing. All stained smears were examined by light microscope x100 lens magnification for the AgNOR quantitation. The NOR mean counts measured by counting the number of silver-stained dots per 20 nucleus for every smear, then the number obtained divided by 20.

Crystal violet stain:

Fixed Smears were stained with 1% crystal violet prepared from stock crystal violet (powder) by distilled water for 1 minute, and then smears were blotted in filter papers and cleared in two changes of Xylene and mounted with DPX medium.

Result interpretation:

Mitotic cells are stained magenta and stand out distinctly against a light blue background of resting cells. Criteria to identify the mitotic cells: the nuclear membrane must be absent, clear, hairy extensions of nuclear material and two parallel or clearly separate chromosome clots. Mitotic figures were observed by light microscope under x 400 magnification. If mitotic figures are present are counted per 1000 buccal cells.

Buccal cell Micronuclei (MNs):

Fixed smears were treated for 1 min each in 50 and 20% ethanol and then washed for 2 min in distilled water. Smears were treated in 5 M hydrochloric acid for 30 minutes and then washed in running tap water for 3 minutes. Smears were drained but not allowed to dry out before being treated in room temperature Schiff's reagent in the dark for 60 minutes. Smears were washed in running tap water for 5 min and rinsed well in distilled water for 1 minute. Smears were stained for 30 seconds in 0.5% light green and rinsed well in distilled water for 2 minutes .Smears were allowed to air-dry, cleared in xylene and mounted in DPX.

Result interpretation:

Nuclei and Micronucleus are stained magenta, while the cytoplasm appears green. Slides were scored using a light microscope at x1000 magnification. Micronuclei were scored only in buccal with uniformly stained nuclei. Cells with condensed chromatin or karyorrhectic cells were not scored for MNs. A total of 1000 buccal cells were scored in order to determine the frequency of MNs in a total of 1000 cells. All data was analyzed by SPSS (statistic package of social science) computer program. Pearson Chi square test was used with 95% confidence level.

CHAPTER FIVE

Results

This is a retrospective case control cohort study assessed oral epithelia proliferative activity by different cytological methods among 210 individuals (100 Toombak users ,100 non-tobacco users and 10 oral cancer patients as an internal control) their ages ranging from 16 to 94 years with a mean age 33 years old. The mean age for the cases was (34 years); hence, the mean age for the controls was (32 years). Seventy one percent of the study populations were below 36 years old, as shown in Table (1).

Table (2) and Figure (1) showing the distribution of the study populations by exposure and age. Age distribution was relatively similar among the two groups in all ranges. Cytological atypia was identified among four (4%) Toombak users and not found in control group, of the four cases with cytological atypia, only one case was identified with moderate degree of cytological atypia and the remaining three were categorized as having mild degree of cytological atypia, as shown in Table (3). All cases with cytological atypia were present in age group more than 36 years old and duration more than 21years, as shown in Table 5. Thirty two (32%) subjects from the cases were identified with keratinization, hence only two subjects from the control groups were identified with keratinization,as shown in Table (3),Figure (2) and photomicrograph (). Toombak dipping is a major factor for occurrence of the keratinization in the oral mucosa. This was found to be statistically significant P < 0.0001.

In regard to the inflammation, 13(13%) and two (2%) of the subjects are indentified with inflammation in cases and control groups respectively, as shown in Table (3) and

Figure(3) .Cases were more susceptible for inflammatory conditions than controls and this was found to be statistically significant P < 0.003.

In regard to the infection, 21(21%) and four (4%) of the cases were identified with bacteria and monilia, respectively, since three (3%) of the control group identified with bacteria, as shown in Table (3), Figure (4) and photomicrograph (). Cases were more susceptible for infections than controls and this was found to be statistically significant P < 0.0001.

The mean NOR counts for cases and controls were 2.423 and1.303 respectively. The mean NOR count was higher in the cases group than control groups, this was found to be statistically significant P < 0.0001, as indicated in table 3.

The mean of the micronuclei frequency per 1000 buccal cells for the cases 1.026 and the control groups 0.356, the micronuclei frequencies was higher in the cases group than control groups. This was found to be statistically significant P < 0.0001.

As indicated in table 5 the mean of NOR count was found to increase with the increasing of duration of exposure and this was found to be statistically significant p< 0.0001 and the relationship between the mean NOR count and the frequency of Toombak use (times per day). The mean NOR count was found to increase with the increasing of the frequency of Toombak use and was found to be statistically significant p<0.001.

In regard to the distribution of the micronuclei frequencies by duration of exposure. There was increasing in the micronuclei frequencies with the increase of exposure duration and this was found to be statistically significant p<0.0001 and There was increasing in micronuclei frequency with the increase of frequency of Toombak use (times per day) and this was found to be statistically significant p<0.001. As indicated in Table 5.

As shown in table (5) the relationship between the amount of Toombak dipped and the proliferative markers (the mean NOR count and micronuclei frequency), there was increasing in the mean NOR count in those snuffing large amount of Toombak per dipp. This was found to be relatively statistically significant; p<0.062 hence There was no relationship between the amount of Toombak dipped and micronuclei frequency; p< 0.866.

As shown in table (5) there was a relationship between the inflammation presence and the mean NOR counts .There was increasing in the mean NOR count in the presence of inflammation. This was found to be statistically significant p<0.006. There was no evidence of relationship between cytological atypia and the presence of inflammation. In regard to the relationship between the inflammation presence and micronuclei frequency. There was no relationship between inflammation presence and micronuclei frequency; p<0.606. There was no association between the type of infection and the proliferative markers (the mean NOR count and micronuclei frequency).

As indicated in Table (5) the relationship between the keratinization presence and the mean NOR count. The highest mean NOR count was associated with keratinization. This was found to be statistically significant; p<0.0001 and the relationship between the keratinization presence and micronuclei frequency. There was a relationship, the higher micronuclei frequencies were identified with keratinization; this was found to be statistically significant; p<0.0001.

In regard to the relationship between the cytological atypia and the proliferative markers (the mean NOR count and micronuclei frequency).The four (100%) cases that showing cytological atypia were demonstrated with mean NOR count more than 2.1and micronuclei frequency more than 2.1.This was found to be statistically significant in micronuclei frequency; $p<0.0001$ and relatively significant in the mean NOR count; $P= 0.134$, as indicated in Table (4).

In regard to the relationship between the age group and proliferative markers (the mean NOR count and micronuclei frequency), there was increasing in the mean NOR count and micronuclei frequency with the age .this was found to be statistically significant $p<0.001$, as shown in Table (4).

As shown in Table (4) the relationship between the age group and the keratinization, inflammation and infection. The keratinization was increasing with increase in the age and this was found to be statistically significant; $p<0.0001$, hence no evidence of relationship between the age group with inflammation and infection.

For the oral cancer patients (internal control); the mean of AgNOR counts and micronuclei frequency was 5.640 and 3.380 respectively. In regard to the mitotic figure presence, the mitotic figure was observed only in the internal control with mean counts 5.530 per 1000 cells. Neither cases groups nor normal control groups were found with mitotic figures.

Table (1): Distribution of the study population by the age.

Age group	Frequency	Percent	Cumulative Percent
<20 years	22	11	11
21-25	54	27	38
26-30	41	20.5	58.5
31-35	24	12	70.5
36+	59	29.5	100.0
Total	200	100	

Table (2): Distribution of the study population by exposure and age.

Age group	Study subjects		
	Cases	Control	Total
< 20 years	9	13	22
21-25	26	28	54
26-30	22	19	41
31-35	11	13	24
36+	32	27	59
Total	100	100	200

Table 3: Distribution of the study population by presence of atypia, keratinization,

inflammation, infection, mean NOR count and micronuclei frequency.

Variable	Category	Cases		Control		P value	RR
		Number	Percent	Number	Percent		Relative risk
Atypia	Mild	3	3%	0	0	0.04	4
	moderate	1	1%	0	0		
	Absent	96	96%	100	100%		
Keratinization presence	Present	32	32%	2	2%	0.0001	16
	Absent	68	68%	98	98%		
Inflammation presence	Present	13	13%	2	2%	0.003	6.5
	Absent	87	87%	98	98%		
Infection presence	Absent	75	75%	97	97%	0.0001	8.3
	Bacteria	21	21%	3	3%		
	Monilia	4	4%	0	0%		
Mean NOR count	Mean	2.423		1.303		0.001	-
Micronuclei frequency	Mean	1.026		0.356		0.001	-

Table 4: The relationship between the proliferative markers(NOR and MNI)

and duration,frequency of Toombak,cytological atypia,inflammation and keratinization.

variable	category	Mean NOR count		Micronuclei frequency			P value
		<2	2.1+	<1	1.1-2	2.1+	
Duration	< 10 years	25	19	37	7	0	NOR P= 0.0001
	11-20	8	20	16	10	2	MNI p= 0.0001
	21+	2	26	6	10	12	
Frequency of	< 20 times/day	14	4	17	1	0	NOR P= 0.0001
Toombak use	21-30	9	27	23	5	8	MNI p= 0.0001
	31-40	2	6	4	4	0	
	41+	10	28	15	17	6	
Amount of	Small	7	19	16	6	4	NOR P= 0.062
Toombak dipped	large	28	46	43	21	10	MNI P= 0.866
per times							
Inflammation	Absent	126	59	147	26	12	NOR P= 0.006
	present	5	10	11	2	2	MNI P=0.606
Keratinization	Absent	119	47	144	15	7	NOR P= 0.0001
	present	12	22	14	13	7	MNI p= 0.0001
Cytological atypia	Absent	35	61	59	27	10	NOR p= 0.134
	present	0	4	0	0	4	MNI p= 0.0001

Table 5: The relationship between the age group and the atypia, keratinization, inflammation, infection, mean NOR count and micronuclei frequency.

Age group	Cytological atypia		keratinzation		Inflammation		Infection		NOR Mean count		Micronuclei frequencies		
	NO	%	NO	%	NO	%	NO	%	<2	2.1+	<1	1.1-2	2.1+
< 20	0	0	0	0	1	6.7%	2	7.1%	21	1	22	0	0
21-25	0	0	5	14.7%	4	26.7%	7	25%	42	12	47	7	0
26-30	0	0	4	11.8%	3	20%	7	25%	45	16	34	6	1
31-35	0	0	5	14.7%	1	6.7%	1	3.6%	16	8	22	2	0
36+	4	100%	20	58.8%	6	40%	11	39.3%	27	32	33	13	13
Total	4	100%	34	100%	15	100%	28	100%	35	65	158	28	14
P value	0.065		0.0001		0.866		0.435		0.0001		0.0001		

Figure (1): Description of the study population by exposure and age

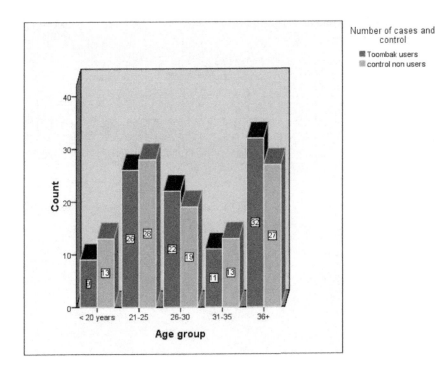

Figure (2): Description of the study population by presence of keratinization

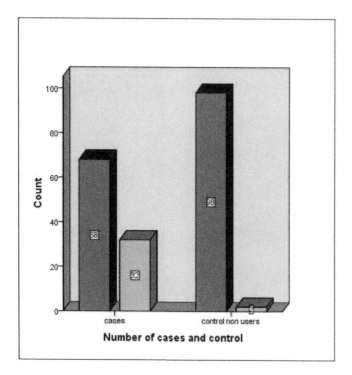

Figure (3): Description of the study population by presence of inflammation

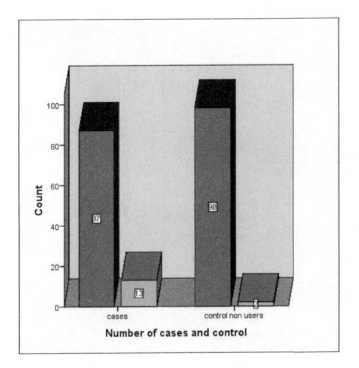

Figure 4: Description of the study population by presence of infection

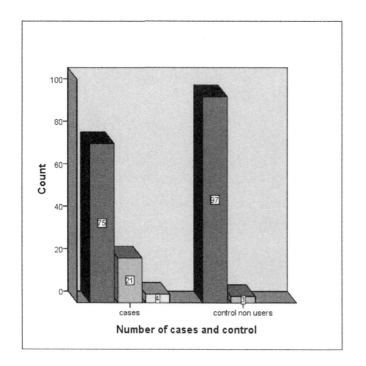

type of infection
■ absent
▨ bacteria
□ monilia

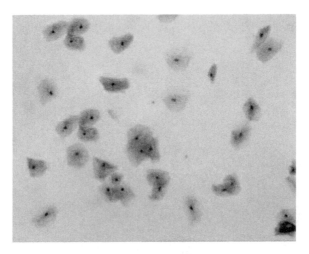

Photomicrograph 1:Normal Buccal Mucosa from Non-tobacco user (Pap stain 40 X)

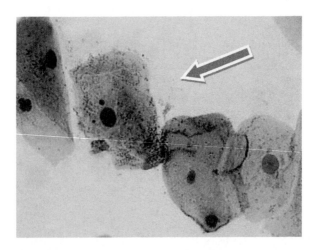

Photomicrograph 2: buccal smear from Toombak user showing bacteria inside the buccal cell (Pap. Stain 100 X).

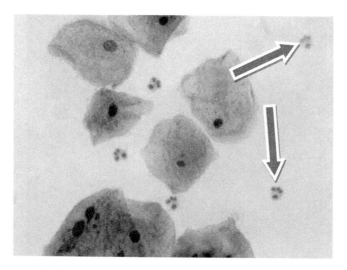

Photomicrograph 3:Buccal smear from Toombak user showing inflammatory cells (Pap. Stain 100 X).

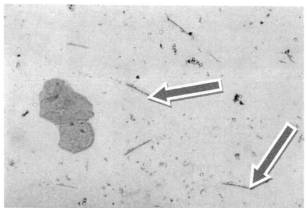

Photomicrograph 4:Buccal smear from toombak user showed a Monilia (Pap. Stain 100 X).

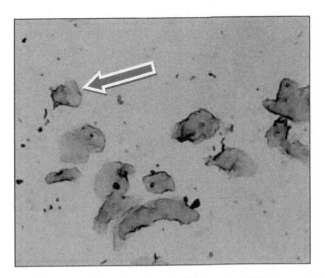

Photomicrograph 5 :Buccal cells from the dipping area showing the keratinization. Anucleated cells appeared in the field (Pap stain 100 X).

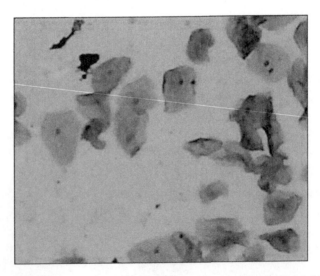

Photomicrograph6: Normal Buccal cells stained with 1% crystal violet (100 X)

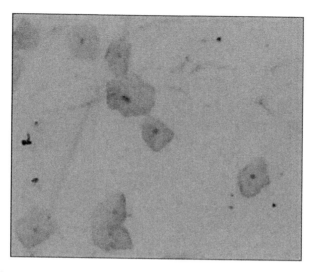

Photomicrograph 7: Normal Buccal cells stained with 1% crystal violet (100 X)

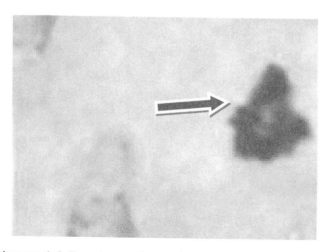

Photomicrograph 8: Buccal smear from oral cancer patient showing mitotic figure nucleus (1% crystal violet 400 x)

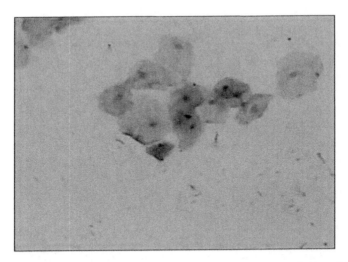

Photomicrograph 9: Normal buccal cells stained by feulogen technique (100 x)

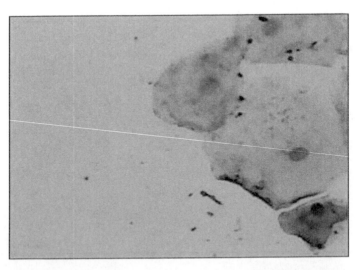

Photomicrograph 10:Normal buccal cells stained by feulogen technique (100 X)

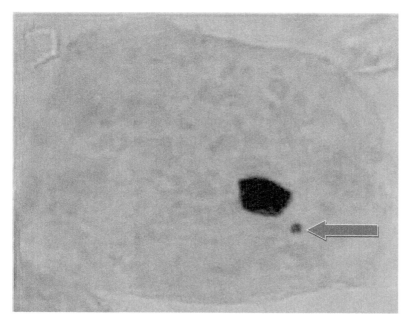

Photomicrograph 11: A buccal cell containing micronuclei small dot beside the nucleus (feulogen technique 400 X)

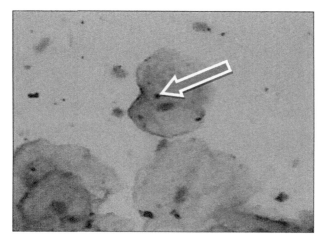

Photomicrograph 12:A Buccal cell containing micronuclei from THE dipping area (feulogen technique 100 x)

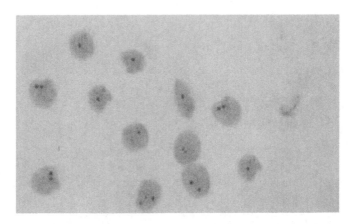

Photomicrograph 13: buccal cells from non tobacoo user stained by AgNOR technique (AgNOR staining 1000 x)

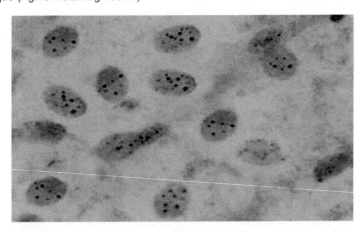

Photomicrograph 14: buccal cells from Toombak user showing more than 5 dots per nucleus (AgNOR staining 1000 x)

CHAPTER SIX

Discussion

Oral cancer is one of the most common cancers worldwide. In Sudan the use of Toombak plays a significant role in etiology of oral squamous cell carcinoma (osccs), with the tobacco specific nitrosamines present in Toombak possibly acting as principal carcinogens (Ahmed and Mahgoob, 2007). For the Screening and early detection of the premalignant and malignant lesions in high-risk groups, simple, reliable and cost-effective screening methods are urgently needed. In this study the four cases found with cytological atypia (dyskaryosis) was identified only in Toombak users. The use of toombak was previously reported to induce cytological atypia and premalignant changes of the oral cavity (Ahmed, et al. 2003). They applied Exfoliative cytology (EFC) to a retrospective cohort to assess the presence and severity of oral epithelial atypia (ET) in 300 subjects (100 toombak dippers; 100 cigarette smokers; 100 non-tobacco users) without prior knowledge of the subjects' tobacco exposure. Five patients with oral squamous cell carcinoma (OSCC) were included as internal controls. ET was ascertained in 29 subjects and could not be ascertained in the remaining 271. Among the 29 subjects with ET, there were 11 (38%) toombak dippers, 14 (48%) cigarette smokers and 4 (14%) non-tobacco users. Among the 271 subjects without ET, there were 89 (33%) toombak dippers, 86 (32%) cigarette smokers and 96 (35%) non-tobacco users. ET was found in all the 5 control cases with OSCC. For the ET among toombak dippers and cigarette smokers, adjusted OR and the 95% CI were found to be 3 (0.91-9.7) and 4 (1.2-12.3), respectively. In the sudan, the high incidence of OSCCs

59

and an equal high prevalence of potentially malignant oral mucosal lesions has been strongly attributed to the habit of toombak use (Idris, *et al.* 1995).

Thirty two (32%) subjects from the cases in this study were identified with keratinization. Since keratinization with anucleation may lead to premalignant lesion called leukoplakia, there is a strong association between cancers of the oral cavity and pharynx and Toombak use. Use of toombak has been showed to produce a variety of oral mucosal changes such as dysplasia and hyperkeratosis (Idris, *et al.* 1996). The keratinization is direct propotion with increase in the age of the cases and this due to prolonged exposure to the Toombak. In regard to the infections and inflammatory conditions, cases were more susceptible than controls, and this was found to be statistically significant. The Erosions and exposure of oral mucosa to the toombak irritating substances are the major causative factors.

The cases group has significantly higher AgNOR mean counts than control group and this indicate there is increase in cellular proliferation in Toombak dippers.this findings supported by the study aimed to assess cellular proliferative activity of clinically healthy oral mucosal epithelial cells of Toombak dippers and smokers by means of AgNOR counts and nuclear areas via nuclear morphometry. Smears were collected from normal-appearing mouth floor mucosa and tongue of 75 toombak dippers, 75 smokers and 50 non-tobacco users between the ages of 20 and 70 with a mean age of 36 years. AgNORs were counted in the first 50 well-fixed, nucleated squamous cells and nuclear areas were calculated via microscopic stage micrometer. Cytological atypia was ascertained in 6 tobacco users and could not be ascertained in non-tobacco users. Statistically mean AgNOR numbers per nucleus in the non-tobacco users (2.45±0.30) was lower than the toombak dippers (3.081±0.39, $p<0.004$), and the smokers (2.715±0.39, $p<0.02$), and mean nuclear areas of epithelial cells of toombak dippers (6.081±0.39, $p<0.009$) and smokers (5.68±10.08, $p<0.01$) was also significantly higher than non-smokers (5.39±9.4). The mean number of nuclei having more than 3 AgNORs was 28%, 19% and 7% in toombak dippers, smokers and non-tobacco users, respectively. These findings support the view that toombak dipping and smoking are severe risk factors for oral mucosal proliferative lesions and exfoliative cytology is valid for screening of oral mucosal lesions (Ahmed and babiker, 2009). The duration, frequency and amount of Toombak use are direct proportion with the AgNOR mean counts and this was found statistically significant. The prolonged exposure of Toombak with frequent large amount is the major causative factors to increase the AgNOR mean in Toombak dippers. The AgNOR mean counts are increased with the presence of keratinization. Kertinization is significant factor to increase the AgNOR counts. There are association between the higher AgNOR mean counts and the inflammation presence and this was found to be statistically significant $p<0.006$. The inflammatory process can cause increasing in the mean AgNOR counts of the cases. This supported by the study; immunohistochemical expression of PCNA and Ki-67 proteins and the histochemical expression of AgNORs were studied in 20 odontogenic keratocysts in order to assess the relationship between epithelial cell proliferation and inflammation within the capsule. A statistically significant increase of PCNA[+] and Ki-67[+] cells and of AgNOR numbers was detected in the linings of inflamed odontogenic keratocysts compared to non-inflamed lesions. The results suggest the existence of greater proliferative activity in the epithelial cells of inflamed odontogenic keratocysts, which may be associated with the disruption of the typical structure of odontogenic keratocyst linings (Paula, et al. 2000).

The cases have significantly higher micronuclei frequency mean than control group that indicate there are possible toxins in Toombak induce the micronuclei. Didn't find previous studies about the micronuclei in the Toombak dippers. The present study findings supported by the study aimed to evaluate the micronuclei (MN) in buccal mucosa of healthy individuals from southern India, Who were regularly chewing a mixture of betel leaf, areca nut and tobacco. A total of 44 subjects were examined. The study population included 15 chewers, 14 chewers with smoking habit and 15 controls with the mean age of 38.57 ± 0.54, 34.50 ± 0.95, and 33.28 ± 0.89 years, respectively. The mean percentage of MN was 1.90 ± 1.03 in chewers, 2.00 ± 1.12 in chewers with smoking habits and 0.81 ± 0.66 in controls. There was no significant difference between the mean percentages of the two experimental groups. It can be concluded that a mixture of betel leaf, areca nut, and tobacco is unsafe for oral health (Sellappa, et al. 2009). In a study the evaluation of micronuclei in buccal mucosa cells of habitual Maras Powder users (smokeless tobacco) and smokers. Buccal cells of both groups showed a higher frequency of micronuclei than nonusers (non smokers, non chewers) (Ozkul, et al. 1997). The micronuclei frequencies is increasing with increase in the duration and frequency of Toombak use and this was found statistically significant; $p<0.0001$ .frequent use and prolonged exposure of Toombak are significant factors to increase the micronuclei frequencies. The presence of keratinization is associated with higher micronuclei frequencies and the inflammation presence in the oral cavity is not associated with micronuclei frequency.

Results of AgNOR,micronuclei and cytological atypical changes show that cellular proliferation is significantly higher in Toombak users which might attributed to the fact that production of a malignant cell require cell proliferation and DNA activity.

The mitotic figure was not observed in the cases and control groups but observed only in the internal control (oral cancer patients).this finding supported by the study aimed to compare the staining of mitotic cells in haematoxylin and eosin with that in crystal violet and to compare the number of mitotic figures present in normal oral mucosa, epithelial dysplasia and oral squamous cell carcinoma in crystal violet-stained sections with that in H and E-stained sections. No mitotic cells were seen either in the crystal violet-stained or in the H and E-stained sections in ten cases of normal oral mucosa. A statistically significant increase in the mean mitotic count was observed in crystal violet-stained sections of epithelial dysplasia as compared to the H and E-stained sections (p = 0.0327). A similar increase in the mitotic counts was noted in crystal violet-stained sections of oral squamous cell carcinoma as compared to the H and E-stained sections.(p = 0.0443). One per cent crystal violet provides a definite advantage over the H and E-stained sections in selectively staining the mitotic figures (Ankle and Kale, 2007).

CHAPTER SEVEN

Conclusion and recommendations

It's clear that Toombak dipping is high risk factor to increase the cellular proliferative activity and DNA damage in the oral mucosa of the Toombak users. Newer prognosticators like immunohistochemistry, flow cytometry, autoradiography, DNA ploidy measurements are now on the forefront. However, cost and time factors make them less feasible. Properly standardized cytochemical methods with precise use can overcome these problems. The cytochemical methods such as agnor counts and micronuclei frequency is simple and cost-effective methods and highly recommended for the assessment of cellular proliferative activity. Oral exfoliative cytology using Pap smear is useful in evaluation of epithelial atypia which is frequently encountered in premalignant and early malignant oral lesions. We need to establish a panel of cellular proliferative cytological methods to treat the drawback like AgNOR counts which affected by inflammation presence when used alone. We need to standardize the cytological proliferative markers methods that are rapid, inexpensive, quantitative, reproducible, technologically simple, and applicable for monitoring and screening subjects who have been identified as being at high risk for developing oral cancer. The subject is aware of risk markers that have been identified in the clinically normal oral mucosa. Thus, the identification of risk markers of oral cancer may serve as an aid in Toombak dipping cessation.

CHAPTER EIGHT

References

- Ahmed HG, Babiker A A. Assessment of cytological atypia, AgNOR and nuclear area in epithelial cells of normal oral mucosa exposed to toombak and smoking. Rare Tumor 2009; 1 (1): 28 - 30.

- Ahmed HG, Idris A M, Ibrahim SO. Study of oral epithelial atypia among Sudanese tobacco users by exfoliative cytology. Anticancer research 2003; 23: 1943-1945.

- Ahmed HG, Mahgoob RM. Impact of Toombak dipping in the etiology of oral cancer: Gender-exclusive hazard in the Sudan. J Can Res Ther 2007; 3:127-30.

- Ankle MR, Kale AD, Charantimath S, Charantimath S. Comparison of staining of mitotic figures by haematoxylin and eosin-and crystal violet stains, in oral epithelial dysplasia and squamous cell carcinoma. Indian J Dent Res 2007; 18:101-5.

- Axell T, Pindborg JJ, Smith CJ, Van der Waal I. Oral white lesions with special reference to precancerous and tobacco-related lesions. J Oral Pathol Med 1996; 25: 49-54.

- Bancroft J, Gamble D, Marilyn. Theory and practice of Histological techniques. 5th ed. Churiche Livingstone. London 2002; 523-524.

- Boen st.changes in nuclei szqumous epithelial cells in perinicious anemia. acta med scand 1957;159:425-431

- Boldy D, Crocker J, Ayres GJ: Application of the AgNOR method to cell imprints of lymphoid tissue. J Pathol 157:75-79, 1989[Medline]

- Brad W, Neville DDS, Terry A. Oral Cancer and Precancerous Lesions. American Cancer Society 2002; 52 (4): 195.

- Burkitt G, Steven A, Lowe J. Wheater's Basic Histopathology. 3th ed. Churchile Livingstone. London 1996; pp 134-135.

- Colecchia M, Leopardi O: Evaluation of AgNOR count in distinguishing benign from malignant mesothelial cells in pleural fluids. Pathol Res Pract 1992; 166:53-60.

- De Paula A.M.B., Carvalhais J.N., Domingues M.G., Barreto D.C., Mesquita R.A. Cell proliferation markers in the odontogenic keratocyst: effect of inflammation. Journal of Oral Pathology & Medicine 2000; 29(10): pp. 477-482.

- Elbeshir E I, Abeen H A, Idris A M, Abbas K. Snuff dipping and oral cancer in Sudan: A retrospective study. British Journal of Oral and Maxillofacial Surgery 1998; 27 (3): 243-248.

- Epstein JB, Zhang L, Rosin M. Advances in the diagnosis of oral premalignant and malignant lesions. J Can Dent. 2002;68:617–21.

- Feldman JG,Hazan M,Nagarajan M, Kissen B. A case-control investigation of alcohol, tobacco, and diet in head and neck cancer. Prev Med 1975; 4:444–63.

- Freddie B; Jacques F, Isabelle S, Rebecca S. Global Cancer Statistics 2018: GLOBOCAN Estimates of Incidence and Mortality Worldwide for 36 Cancers in 185 Countries. CA CANCER J CLIN 2018;68:394–424.

- Gloeckler Ries LA, Miller BA, Hankey BF, Kosary CL, Harras A, Edwards BK, eds. SEER cancer statistics review, 1973-1991. Bethesda, Md: US Department of Health and Human Services, Public Health Service, National Cancer Institute. Report number NIH-94-2789. 1994.

- Graham S, Dayal H, Rohrer T, et al. Dentition, diet, tobacco and alcohol in the epidemiology of oral cancer. J Natl Cancer Inst 1977; 59:1611–8.

- Greer RO, Eversole S, Crosby LK. Detection of papillomavirus genomic DNA in oral epithelial dysplasias, oral smokeless tobacco associated leukoplakias and epithelial malignancy. Journal of Oral Maxillofac Surgery 1990; 48:1201-5.

- Hazare VK, Goel RR, Gupta PC (1998) Oral submucous fibrosis, areca nut and pan masala use: a case-control study. Natl Med J India 11, 299

- Hoffman D, Djordjevic MV, Fan J. Five leading US commercial brands of moist snuff in 1994: assessment of carcinogenic N-nitrosamines. J Natl Cancer Inst 1995; 87:1862-9.

- Idris Ali M, Ibrahim Y E, Warnakulasuriya K A A S, Cooper D J, Johnson N. Toombak Use and Cigarette Smoking in the Sudan: Estimates of Prevalence in the Nile State. American Health Foundation and Academic Press 1998; 27(4): 597–603.

- Idris AM, Prokopczyk B, Hoffmann D. Toombak: a major risk factor for cancer of the oral cavity in Sudan. Prev Med 1994;23(6):832-9.

- Idris M, Ahmed H M, Mukhtar B I, Gadir A F, El-Beshir E I. Descriptive epidemiology of oral neoplasms in sudan 1970-1985 and the role of toombak. International Journal of Cancer 1995; 61(2):155 – 158.

- Idris, A. M, WarnakulasuriyaK. A. A. S, Ibrahim Y E, Nielsen R, Cooper D, Johnson N W. Toombak-associated oral mucosal lesions in Sudanese show a low prevalence of epithelial dysplasia. Journal of Oral Pathology & Medicine 1996; 25: 5.

- Jemal A, Siegel R, Ward E, Murray T, Xu J, Smigal C, Thun M. "Cancer statistics, 2006". *CA Cancer J Clin* (2006); 56 (2): 106–30.

- Konopacka M. Effect of smoking and aging on micronucleus frequencies in human exfoliated buccal cells. Neoplasma 2003; 50:380–2.

- Koss, L G. Diagnostic Cytology and its Histopathologic Bases. 5[th]edition. J.B.Lippincott Company, London. 2005; pp 716-720.

- Luo LZ, Werner KM, Gollin SM, Saunders WS. Cigarette smoke induces anaphase bridges and genomic imbalances in normal cells. Mutat Res 2004; 554:375–85.

- Luthere E, Lindner. Improvements in the Silver-staining Technique for Nucleolar Organizer Regions (AgNOR). The Journal of Histochemistry and Cytochemistry 1993; 41 (3): 439-445.

- Mamaev NN, Medvedeva NV, Shust VF, *et al.* Nucleoli and AgNORs in Hodgkin's disease. *J Clin Pathol Mol Pathol* 1997; 50:149–52.

- Mashberg A, Samit A. Early diagnosis of asymptomatic oral and oropharyngeal squamous cancers. CA- A Cancer Journal for Clinicians 1995; 45(6):328-351.

- Mashburg A, Samit AM. Early detection, diagnosis and management of oral and oropharyngeal cancer. CA Cancer J Clin 1989;39:67–88

- Million RR, Cassisi NJ, Mancuso AA. Management of head and neck cancers: a multidisciplinary approach. 2nd ed. J.B. Lippincott. Philadelphia 1994; pp 321-400.

- Murata M, Takayama K, Choi B, Pak A (1996). "A nested case-control study on alcohol drinking, tobacco smoking, and cancer". Cancer Detect Prev 20 (6): 557–65

- Nersesyan, A., Kundi, M., Atefie, K., Schulte-Hermann, R. & Knasmuller, S. Effect of staining procedures on the results of micronucleus assays with exfoliated oral mucosa cells. Cancer Epidemiol. Biomarkers Prev. 15, 1835–1840 (2006).

- Ozkul Y, Donmez H, Erenmemisoglu A, Demirtas H, Imamoglu N. Induction of micronuclei by smokeless tobacco on buccal mucosa cells of habitual users. Mutagenesis 1997; 12:285–7.

- P. Vajdovich, R. Psáder, Z. A. Tóth and E. Perge: Use of the Argyrophilic Nucleolar Region Method for Cytologic and Histologic Examination of the Lymph Nodes in Dogs. Vet Pathol41:338-345 (2004).

- Parkin DM, Bray F, Ferlay J, Pisani P. Global cancer statistics, 2002. CA Cancer J Clin 2005; 55:74–108.

- Patton L L, Epstein J B, Kerr R A. Adjunctive techniques for oral cancer examination and lesion diagnosis: A systematic review of the literature. JADA 2008; 139: 1-2.

- Reshmi SC, Gollin SM. Chromosomal instability and marker chromosome evolution oral squamous cell carcinoma. Genes Chromosomes Cancer 2004;41:38–46.

- Ridge JA, Glisson BS, Lango MN. "Head and Neck Tumors" in Pazdur R, Wagman LD, Camphausen KA, Hoskins WJ (Eds) Cancer Management: A Multidisciplinary Approach. 11 ed. 2008.

- Saunders WS, Shuster M, Huang X, et al. Chromosomal instability and cytoskeletal defects in oral cancer cells. Proc Natl Acad Sci U S A 2000; 97:303–8.

- Shafer WG, Waldron CA. Erythroplakia of the oral cavity. Cancer 1975; 36:1021-8.

- Shulman JD, Beach MM, Rivera-Hidalgo F. The prevalence of oral mucosal lesions in U.S. adults: data from the Third National Health and Nutrition Examination Survey 1988-1994. J Am Dent Assoc 2004; 135:1279–86.

- Silverman S. Oral cancer. 5th ed. American Cancer Society. Hamilton (Ontario, Canada): BC Decker, Inc.; 2003. p. 212.

- Spafford MF, Koch WM, Reed AL, Califano JA, Xu LH, Eisenberger CF, et al. Detection of head and neck squamous cell carcinoma among exfoliated oral mucosal cells by microsatellite analysis. *Clin Cancer Res.* 2001;7:607.

- Stich HF, Curtis JR, Parida BB (1982) Application of the micronucleus test to exfoliated cells of high cancer risk groups: tobacco chewers. Int J Cancer 30, 553-559.

- Sudha Sellappa, Mythili, Sangeetha, Subashini ,Palanisamy.Induction of micronuclei in buccal mucosa on chewing a mixture of betel leaf, areca nut and tobacco. Oral Science 2009; 51(2):289-292.

- Takahashi I,KOBAYASHI TK, Suzuki H. coexistence of pemiphigus vulgaris and herpes virus infection in orla mucosa diagnosed by cytology immune-histochemistry and PCR. Diagn cytopathol 1998;19:440-450

- Taybos G. Oral changes associated with tobacco use. Am J Med Sci 2003; 326:179–82.

- Thomas, P, Harvey, S., Gruner, T. & Fenech, M. The buccal cytome and micronucleus frequency is substantially altered in Down's syndrome and normal ageing compared to young healthy controls. Mutat. Res 2007; 638: 37-47.

- Tolbert, P.E., Shy, C.M. & Allen, J.W. Micronuclei and other nuclear anomalies in buccal smears: methods development. Mutat. Res. 271, 69–77 (1992).

- Torsten W, Remmerbach, Weidenbach H, Müller C, Hemprich A, Pomjanski N, Buckstegge B, Böcking A. Diagnostic value of nucleolar organizer regions (AgNORs) in brush biopsies of suspicious lesions of the oral cavity. Analytical Cellular Pathology 2003; 25 (3): 139-146.

- Zarbo RJ, Crissman JD. The surgical pathology of head and neck cancers. Semin Oncol 1988; 15: 9 -10.

Appendix (1)

Questionnaire

بسم الله الرحمن الرحمن الرحيم
Sudan University for S&T
College of Graduate Studies
Medical Labs Sciences-histo-cytopathology

Questionnaire

Name:... No:.............................

Age :...................................... sex:.....................

Residence:............................. occupation:......................................

Duration of toobmak snuffing:............... snuffing/day:.......................

Amount snuffed/time :

Small ( ) – medium( ) –large ( ) .

Suffer from Chronic diseases: yes ( ) No ()   oral hygiene status:
Good ( ) bad ( ) moderate ().

Presence of other habit affect buccal cavity: yes ( )   NO ( )

If yes mention it:..

Appendix (2)

Materials and instruments used in the collection of the specimens include:

- Sterile wooden tongue depressor
- Disposable gloves.
- Frosted glass slide (75X25X0.2mm)
- Absolute ethyl alcohol.
- Distilled water.

Materials and instruments used in the processing of the specimens include:

- Harris haematoxylin components(Haematoxylin-potassium alum - mercuric oxide-glacial acid).
- Orange G6 component (phosphotungestic acid –orange G).
- EA50(light SF –eosin Y).
- Eosin
- Concentrated hydrochloric HCL.
- Alkaline tap water.
- Xylene (supher free)
- DPX mounting media.
- Gover glass(22X50mm).
- Strong Amonia.
- 95% ethyl alcohol.
- Absolute alcohol 95ml.
- Distilled water 5ml.
- Crystal violet stain
- Silver nitrate
- Sodium thiosulphate
- Gelatin
- Formic acid
- Shiff"s reagent
- Light green stain

Abstract   4

CHAPTER ONE   6

CHAPTER TWO   11

CHAPTER THREE   33

CHAPTER FOUR   34

CHAPTER FIVE   39

CHAPTER SIX   59

CHAPTER SEVEN   64

CHAPTER EIGHT   65

Appendix   72

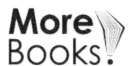
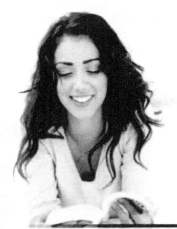
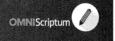

Printed in Great Britain
by Amazon